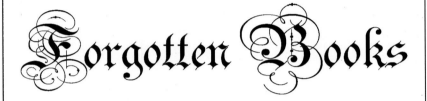

ISBN 978-1-5276-4276-8
PIBN 10877553

This book is a reproduction of an important historical work. Forgotten Books uses state-of-the-art technology to digitally reconstruct the work, preserving the original format whilst repairing imperfections present in the aged copy. In rare cases, an imperfection in the original, such as a blemish or missing page, may be replicated in our edition. We do, however, repair the vast majority of imperfections successfully; any imperfections that remain are intentionally left to preserve the state of such historical works.

1 MONTH OF
FREE
READING

at

www.ForgottenBooks.com

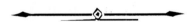

By purchasing this book you are eligible for one month membership to ForgottenBooks.com, giving you unlimited access to our entire collection of over 1,000,000 titles via our web site and mobile apps.

To claim your free month visit:
www.forgottenbooks.com/free877553

English
Français
Deutsche
Italiano
Español
Português

www.forgottenbooks.com

Mythology Photography **Fiction**
Fishing Christianity **Art** Cooking
Essays Buddhism Freemasonry
Medicine **Biology** Music **Ancient**
Egypt Evolution Carpentry Physics
Dance Geology **Mathematics** Fitness
Shakespeare **Folklore** Yoga Marketing
Confidence Immortality Biographies
Poetry **Psychology** Witchcraft
Electronics Chemistry History **Law**
Accounting **Philosophy** Anthropology
Alchemy Drama Quantum Mechanics
Atheism Sexual Health **Ancient History**
Entrepreneurship Languages Sport
Paleontology Needlework Islam
Metaphysics Investment Archaeology
Parenting Statistics Criminology
Motivational

ARMY MEDICAL LIBRARY
FOUNDED 1836

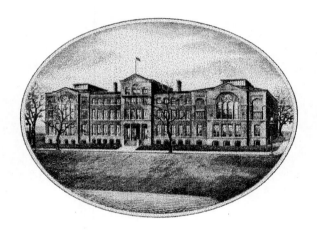

WASHINGTON, D.C.

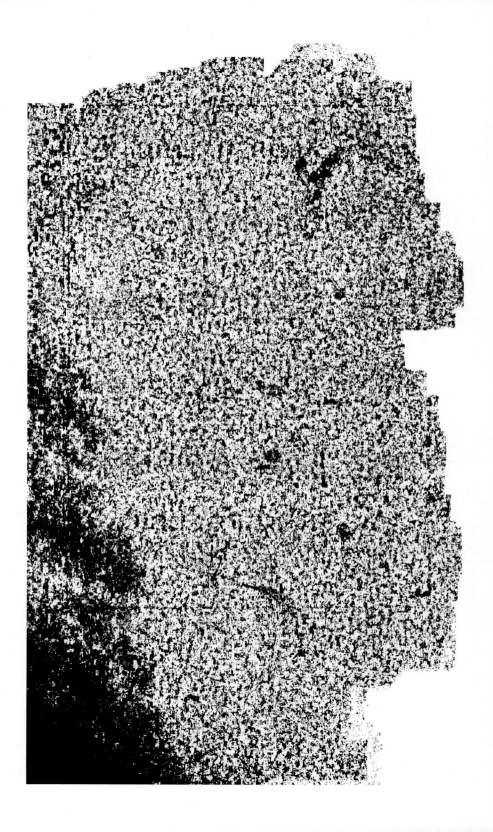

THE USE

OF

BRANDY AND SALT,

AS

A REMEDY

FOR VARIOUS

INTERNAL AS WELL AS EXTERNAL DISEASES,

INFLAMMATION AND LOCAL INJURIES;

CONTAINING

AMPLE DIRECTIONS FOR MAKING AND APPLYING IT.

Illustrated and Explained by the Discoverer,

WILLIAM LEE, Esq.

BOSTON:

C. C. P. MOODY, PRINTER, OLD DICKINSON OFFICE, 52 WASHINGTON ST.

1851.

PREFACE.

By the publication of the following little work, to give increased publicity to the remedy of Brandy and Salt, I am actuated by a desire to benefit my fellow men, and to do what in my power lies to alleviate the distresses of suffering humanity. Having myself experienced the beneficial effects of this simple but powerful remedy, and having seen it in numerous cases prove an antidote to many of the common ills of life, I am most anxious that the good thus effected should be generally known, that the afflicted may have the opportunity of reaping such advantages from it as their respective circumstances may require, believing it, as I do, to be the greatest discovery in medicine in modern times; and its adoption, if not attended by any efficacious results, will yet be accompanied by no deleterious consequences.

This pamphlet, though simple, like the remedy of which it treats, would be as a family book of reference in cases of sickness, in my opinion, one of the most useful ever laid upon a table, and I write from the experience of ten years of the use of this remedy.

☞ *Be sure not to shake the salt up when you use the remedy, as it must be quite clear, and never take it without being diluted in hot water, except for Worms and Paralytic attacks.*

THE USE OF

BRANDY AND SALT,

A REMEDY

FOR VARIOUS INTERNAL AS WELL AS EXTERNAL DISEASES, &c.

USE FRENCH BRANDY ONLY.

THE inquiry has often been made of me whether gin, rum, or spirits of wine, will not do as well as brandy, or if British brandy is not as good as French brandy. With regard to the first three, gin, rum, or spirits of wine, I should recommend all such to make the experiment for themselves; for myself, I have always been content with French brandy. But with regard to whether British brandy is as good as French brandy, I will relate an occurrence which took place in a neighboring town in this county :—Two gentlemen, from the perusal of one of my letters in the Intelligencer, agreed to make use of the remedy, for the same complaint; I believe, the rheumatism. They mixed and used it according to the prescription. After a few days they compared notes, when it was found that one of them was almost cured, whilst the other was not at all better. They then spoke of the manner they had mixed and used it, of the kind of brandy, &c., when it came out that the one cured used French brandy, and the other British brandy. If they had both used British brandy, they would have come to the same conclusion that one of the faculty of Leeds came to when my first letter was published, that what I stated was all lies, but upon much better grounds, though equally untrue. When my first communication was published in the Leeds Intelligencer, it was so pronounced to be ; but as I suppose, this gentleman spoke more by his wishes and his interest, than actual knowledge, though I believe that he is clever in his profession, and a worthy man, I think he ought to be excused ; only it shows the necessity of men being careful before they accuse another of publishing lies, lest, in so doing, they speak untruths themselves. And this brings to my mind a suspicion which is entertained by some as it was spoken of in a society where I was, that as I live in France, and possess an estate there, I recommend it from interested motives, having, no doubt, a manufactory of brandy upon the estate. This idea may have great weight with many, for there are large numbers in society, who, seeing that most things turn upon self-interest, think that it is not possible that any one should act from any thing but interested motives. But to all such I would say, neither my estate, nor the village attached to it, nor the country near it, has, ever since I possessed it, though it is now fifteen years, in all that time produced as much brandy as I give away every week upon an average, one week with another; indeed, it has never produced, I believe, one table-spoonful; therefore, the suspicion that I have ever had any interested motives is erroneous and unjust.

In conclusion, I beg leave to say, that as a remedy it is unrivalled; whether it is used internally or externally, it is equally efficacious, and for both, or either, there cannot be found its equal; therefore, as a remedy, it is almost perfect. As a discovery I cannot but think it stands unrivalled also, at least in medicine, as there is nothing made public which is equal to it as an universal specific. It cures complaints which have hitherto been deemed incurable. This has been thought to be an objection to it; but let these objectors apply it according to the rules laid down in this treatise, and I think they will blush at their want of caution. As a remedy, which is easily made, I do think it cannot be exceeded; all that is wanted is to apply a sufficient quantity of salt to the brandy, shake it together, and it is ready for use as soon as it is clear.

METHOD OF MAKING THE REMEDY.

Half fill a bottle with brandy, and add to it one third the quantity of salt; cork and shake well together. When mixed, let the salt settle to the bottom, and be particularly careful to use it when clear, the clearer the better. Many persons have made a great mistake in shaking it up just before it is used. The efficacy is not near so great, and to open sores the application is much more painful, from the particles of salt which are not dissolved in the brandy; but the salt and brandy should remain together, and when all the brandy is used off more may be added to the salt. Though it is ready for use in twenty minutes after it is put together, it is good at any time after; and it is a perfect medicine, as it has the rare quality of being greatly efficacious in either internal or external application.

GENERAL RULES TO BE OBSERVED IN USING THE REMEDY.

Begin with taking one table-spoonful, mixed in a little hot water or tea, an hour before breakfast, and gradually increase, if the stomach will bear it, to two. The remedy must always be taken in water as hot as the patient can drink it, except in cases of worms and paralytic attacks, and in those two cases to be taken pure.

For children from two to ten years of age, one half of the quantity here prescribed will be sufficient, and increase it according to the age above those years.

In all cases where the head is directed to be rubbed, it should be done so all over, from the back to the front, and the hair made very wet, with the remedy pure; the more hair the better. The operation should be continued for ten minutes or a quarter of an hour before going to bed, and the head should then be covered with the cap only. For pain in any part of the body except the head, bind the parts affected with linen saturated with the remedy.

Abstinence from Intoxicating Drinks.—To insure success it is absolutely necessary that, during its application, whether internally or externally, the patient should strictly abstain from all stimulating and exciting drinks, except the Brandy and Salt. This is a rule which can never be departed from with safety.

Opening Medicine.—The bowels must be kept open at all times, but especially when the patient is using the remedy. The kind of opening medicine which I recommend and use myself, as I find it answers best, is the following :—Four ounces of Epsom salts, dissolved in half a pint of hot water ; then add half a pint of cold water and one tea-spoonful of the essence of peppermint. A wine-glassful to be taken when required, on going to bed. It is better to add half a table-spoonful of brandy to each dose.

I subjoin the following as the line of conduct I followed in my own case, and which I extract from my former pamphlet, published in October, 1839, as it may be of considerable service.

I found it very efficacious to wet a piece of fine linen with the remedy, and bind it on my leg, which I kept moist by pouring a few drops on the linen ; the more frequently I did so the better. This I strictly attended to for about three weeks, and though my leg had been very bad for many months, and bid defiance to the best medical aid I could procure, which caused me to give up all hopes of recovery, to my great surprise the inflammation was entirely gone, the wounds healed, and the leg well in a month. This I publish for the benefit and encouragement of the afflicted, as the cure it wrought upon me was so astonishing to myself and others ; had not this been the case, this pamphlet would never have been re-published by me ; but with great gratitude to the Giver of all good, and thanks to the discoverer, I have complied with his request in making it as public as possible, both by newspaper and pamphlet. I am glad to hear and to see that this remedy is doing good to numbers, for both internal and external complaints. Any person receiving benefit from the application, would do well to let me know, as it may stimulate others; but let no one expect to be cured without perseverance.

DISEASES AND MODE OF TREATMENT.

DIZZINESS IN THE HEAD is cured by washing the crown of the head with the remedy pure. It ought to be rubbed for half an hour, even when the dizziness is removed. Sometimes it feels cured during the operation ; sometimes in an hour after ; and even it has not been removed until after retiring to bed. There are instances of this complaint returning several times, but it is easily subdued by the manner of applying this remedy.

DETERMINATION OF BLOOD TO THE HEAD, which, by the regular mode of practice is sought to be cured by bleeding with leeches about the temples, though it does not always cure, generally brings the patient to the borders of the grave. This complaint is greatly abated, and very often cured, by rubbing the crown of the head with the remedy. Sometimes it is removed very soon, and generally by one operation; if not, it may be repeated once, in which case it is necessary that the afflicted should take two table-spoonsful of the remedy, diluted with six or eight table-spoonsful of hot water. The rubbing of the head is always the best on retiring to bed, and the dose should be taken in the morning, about an hour before breakfast, and repeated several times.

HEADACHES are removed by rubbing the head with the remedy, in the same manner as for Determination of Blood to the Head. I have applied it in hundreds of instances, and always with success; but in case the Headache proves obstinate, it should be repeated, and two table-spoonsful, with six or eight table-spoonsful of hot water, should be taken; but it is generally cured by rubbing once.

INFLAMMATION IN THE EYES.—Before I speak of the manner in which it is cured, I would say, that this remedy, if it only cured this complaint in the manner it does, is beyond all price. There is no occasion for dark rooms; no occasion to desist from the ordinary occupations of the afflicted; no cauterizing of the eye, which very often causes the afflicted to lose their sight; no distress in families. It is cured by the patient wetting the corner of his handkerchief five or six times each day, with the remedy, pure, when he is at his work, when he is walking, when he is riding, when he is buying or selling his merchandize; and rubbing it each time well into his eye. The pain is very trifling, and the cure certain. How different this is from the usual treatment. A friend of mine was shut up in a dark room for ten weeks. He had his eye cauterized several times, besides having several operations performed upon him, and after all his eye is not so well cured as it would have been by this remedy in a fortnight, if it had been taken in time; but in that case he perhaps would have said the inflammation was not severe.

INFLAMMATION OF THE EYES.—The eye to be bathed two or three times a day with a portion of the remedy diluted in an equal quantity of water. If the eye be much inflamed, add a white bread poultice on going to bed, placed between two cloths.

INFLAMMATION IN THE BRAIN is cured by rubbing the crown of the head with the remedy until the pain is removed. There are several instances in which very valuable lives might have been prolonged by the use of this remedy. Malibran, whilst at Manchester, fell a sacrifice to it ; and I am confident that if it had been applied as above, her life would have been spared.

TOOTHACHE is cured in a manner which I discovered myself. It is simply by filling the ear on that side of the head where the pain is with the remedy pure, and letting it remain in the ear for ten minutes, in most cases sufficient to remove the pain. I have seldom known it fail. For any other than decayed teeth the cure is generally permanent. For decayed teeth it may return again upon taking cold ; it should remain in the ear from five to ten minutes.

EARACHE is cured the same as the Toothache, by filling the ear with the remedy. This is rather a pleasant operation, and calculated to do great good in other respects.

DEAFNESS is greatly relieved, and very often cured, by the same method, filling the ear with the remedy. I have known it to be of great use in several instances ; and since I have filled my ears with it I can hear with greater clearness. The best time is upon retiring to rest. Fill first the ear which is the least affected with deafness, and let it remain in for ten minutes ; after which fill the other ear, and let it remain in the ear all night. It conduces very much to sound sleeping.

TEETH ARE PRESERVED by putting a little of the remedy, once each week or fortnight, upon the tooth brush when it is used. This will also remove any soreness which may be in the teeth from eating sour fruit, or any other cause.

GUM BOILS are cured by saturating a piece of fine linen with the remedy, and applying it to the part, betwixt the gums and the cheek. The best time is upon retiring to rest, and letting it remain the whole of the night ; this will remove the most violent pain. But the same operation requires to be repeated several nights to remove the boil and prevent the teeth from becoming loose.

ERUPTIONS UPON THE FACE AND HEAD are generally removed by rubbing the part with the remedy. If they are of a cancerous nature, and of a few weeks' standing, the remedy gives no pain, and the cure is effected with surprising facility ; but to all other descriptions of eruptions it gives pain.

AGUE, OR INTERMITTING FEVERS, are cured by rubbing the head once, on retiring to rest, and next morning taking two table-spoonsful, diluted with six table-spoonsful of hot water for a man, and half the quantity for a female, an hour before breakfast. It should be repeated for twelve mornings, or until the disorder is subdued.

CHOLIC is generally cured in four or five minutes, by taking two table-spoonsful of the remedy, diluted with hot water. If it is not cured by the first operation, it ought to be repeated, and the dose made stronger. It seldom requires repeating more than twice, though I have known it repeated three times.

CHOLERA is cured by rubbing the head once or twice, or as often as the pains in the head return, and by taking two or three table-spoonsful, diluted with hot water. This should be repeated several times each day, if the attack is very strong, at short intervals; and if the skin is discolored, the part ought to be rubbed with it until the complaint is subdued, which will be known by the removal of the pain.

QUINSEY, OR SORE THROATS, should be grappled with in every possible way, first by gargling with the remedy pure, second by fill-ing each ear with the remedy pure, one after the other, and letting it remain in each ear ten minutes. I have found great relief from this method, and the best time is upon retiring to rest. Then a little linen, saturated with the remedy, should be wrapped round the neck, and kept moist ; these methods are generally successful ; but if not the danger from the sore throat becoming something worse is greatly reduced. This is one of those complaints which require great per-severance, and even the use of leeches may be necessary after all ; but such cases will be very rare.

INFLAMMATION IN THE BOWELS is cured by taking two table-spoonsful of the remedy, diluted with hot water, repeatedly, and at short intervals, until the pain is removed. It is also well to rub the exterior, and apply warm flannel to the part, which may be kept warm, or even hot, by applying a warming pan to the flannel. I have found great benefit from this operation.

PAINS IN THE SIDE, which are often the forerunners of Pleurisies and other Fevers. After the crown of the head has been rubbed, the side should be well rubbed with the remedy until the pain is re-moved. If this does not succeed, it will be necessary to take a piece of linen, about half a yard square, and double it several times, until it becomes six inches square ; saturate it well with the remedy, and apply it to the part ; it should be kept moist. It has been of great use in numberless instances, and generally removes the pain in less than an hour, and very often prevents fever. It will also be well for the patient to take two table-spoonsful of the remedy, diluted with hot water.

RHEUMATISM is always relieved, and often cured, by rubbing with this remedy upon the part afflicted. But it ought to be contin-ued for several days, or even weeks, once or twice each day, and there are cases in which it is necessary the patient should take two table-spoonsful, mixed with hot water, once a day, for twelve or four-teen days. This is one of the most stubborn complaints in existence, and requires great patience and perseverance ; but even this has been obliged to yield to the remedy, though the use of a brush is sometimes necessary. A great many instances might be adduced of persons afflicted with this complaint who have been obliged to pass their winters, in great pain, within doors, but by its application have been able to enjoy themselves during the whole of the year.

GOUT AND RHEUMATIC GOUT.—These painful disorders being in the blood, it will be necessary that the person afflicted should have his or her crown of the head well rubbed with the remedy, once, on retiring to rest; the morning after take two table-spoonsful mixed with hot water, an hour before breakfast, which should be repeated for twelve or fourteen days, and the part inflamed, or where the pain is, touched with something soft, perhaps a feather, until the patient can bear to rub it with the finger. These are complaints which require great perseverance.

GRAVEL.—Take a table-spoonful (diluted) three or four times a day.

BURNS AND SCALDS are very soon cured by this remedy. The part affected should be rubbed with the pure liquid. The first application is painful, but not of long continuance, and each application is less painful. The sore is soon cured, but sometimes it is necessary to apply something to soften the sore; tallow or hog's lard is good, or anything else of a softening nature.

CHILBLAINS are cured by the application of this remedy; but care should be taken that the part affected should be rubbed until perfectly dry. There is also another cure, which is simply washing the hands or feet in a strong ley of salt and water, and let it dry upon them.

INSANITY, OR WHAT IS CALLED AFFECTION OF THE NERVES, which produces lowness of spirits, may be almost always prevented by rubbing the crown of the head twice or thrice with this remedy. But it ought to be well rubbed each time for ten minutes, or a quarter of an hour; and I think, in order to confirm the cure, two table-spoonsful should be taken for twelve mornings, fasting, diluted with hot water. Children of the age of four years, and under, are cured by rubbing the crown of the head only once. I have had so many proofs of it that I can speak with great confidence. There is only one case in which it was not successful, and that was an eruption on the skin; in all other complaints, whether illness or weakness, it has been successful. There are many instances in the village near my castle; and those children are far more healthy and handsome than those who have not had their heads rubbed with the remedy. I happened to call at one of my farms, and found three children in the ague; they were in a state of great prespiration: the eldest was nine years old; the other two under three; they were all rubbed upon the crown of the head. During the operation every one was better, and before I left the house they appeared free from pain. I did not see them after, but I inquired very often, and their father said they had never had any return of the fever. The surprising effects of this remedy, from rubbing the crown of the head, particularly in infants, lead me to doubt the generally received opinion that headaches are caused by the state of the stomach; and I am convinced, by observation, that the state of the head not only acts upon the stomach, but upon all other parts of the human frame. This, I think, has been a mistake among professional men; and no doubt they will be offended at me for venturing to question the generally received opinion; but as my opinions are founded upon close observation and facts, I beg of them to turn their attention (with a proper allowance that even the most generally received ideas may be erroneous) to the investigation of this great truth. But let them come to what conclusion they may, they cannot throw a doubt upon the fact that children are cured by rubbing the crown of the head with this remedy.

CANCERS.—I have had such great success in the cure of them that I thought it never failed, and that merely by rubbing or washing the sore. There are at present some doubts whether it cures those of a very long standing or not, but there is not the least doubt that it will cure those which have been in existence for a year, and it may be easily known whether the sore is of a cancerous nature or not by the application of the remedy. If it is so, the application gives no pain, and the cure is rapid; to all other sores it gives pain. For cancers of long standing, I recommend that the crown of the head should be well rubbed with the remedy, and that the patient should take two table-spoonsful, diluted with hot water every morning. The sore ought to be washed with the remedy, and soft linen saturated with the remedy applied, and kept, if possible, constantly to it. In all cases, if this method is followed, it will be a great relief, and generally a cure; and, for the future, there will be very few bad cancers, if the remedy is applied in their early stage.

WORMS.—Take two table-spoonsful of the remedy pure, an hour before breakfast; for a child, from five to seven years of age, half the quantity is sufficient.

FEVERS.—In all cases of fever, and there are several kinds, rubbing the crown of the head with the remedy should be the very first operation, and immediately after the patient should take two table-spoonsful, diluted with hot water; this should be repeated at intervals of from an hour to three hours, according to the nature and violence of the attack. No amendment can be hoped for until the inflammation is reduced, and nothing will reduce it so soon as this remedy, and that without bleeding and blistering; but all complaints are the most easily cured at their commencement.

INFLAMMATION ON THE LUNGS will generally be relieved by

washing the crown of the head, and taking two table-spoonsful, diluted with hot water. But it should be taken several times each day, and a piece of linen, several thicknesses, saturated with the remedy, put upon the part where the pain is.

C_{ONSUM}^P_{TIONS}.—I have not the least doubt but the majority might be cured by an application of this remedy, in its earlier stages, and that without confinement, by first rubbing the crown of the head once, and taking one or two table-spoonsful of the remedy, diluted with hot water, every morning, an hour before breakfast; it will be well to rub the chest once each morning. There are two cases of its almost wonderful effects, one at La Ferté Imbault, and the other in the Isle of Man.* As the remedy is a new discovery, the cases of its cure of this complaint are not many; but only let it be properly and generally used, and I have no doubt but millions will derive benefit from it each year.

ASTHMAS are greatly relieved by rubbing the crown of the head once, before retiring to rest, and taking one or two table-spoonsful diluted with hot water, for several mornings. The sister of the curate of our Parish, in France, had been long afflicted with asthma, and, after repeated recommendations, she had been induced to try it; her brother always said, to any inquiry, that she was well since she had used the remedy, therefore I hope that it will do good in all cases, and cure in some.

COLDS AND COUGHS are greatly relieved by the application of this remedy to the parts affected. If in the head, the head should be rubbed; if in the throat, the ears should be filled, one after the other, and let remain for ten minutes, the throat gargled, and the neck and breast rubbed with the remedy. They are oft very tedious, and require great perseverance, and even with all this it is ne-

* BRANDY AND SALT.—Our last number contained a long account of a novel yet simple medicine, (a mixture of brandy and salt) strongly recommended by its discoverer, as a powerful remedy in several dangerous maladies which afflict the human race. As the article in question was not the puff for a quack nostrum; but written by a gentleman with a view to benefit his fellow creatures, we readily gave it insertion, and are now glad of having been the means of increasing its publicity, as we have since had an opportunity of witnessing its efficacy in a case wherein the life of the patient seemed to be in imminent peril. A young man, who had resided for some time in this Island, went to South Carolina three years ago with the intention of settling in that state, where all his friends reside: but a southern climate not agreeing with his constitution, he returned to Douglas about a month since, apparently labouring under a confirmed consumption, in the hope of benefiting under a change of air. Having read a description of the above named medicine, he began to give it a trial, and after persevering according to the prescription for nearly three weeks, all the consumptive symptoms vanished, and he became so greatly improved both in health and appearance, that he is now actually preparing for his return to America; but with the design of fixing in a more salubrious part of that flourishing country.—*Manx Liberal.*

cessary to apply leeches. If the chest is attacked, the patient should apply a piece of soft linen, of several thicknesses, to the breast, saturated with the remedy, and kept moist. The effects of this application is sometimes very striking.

DYSENTERY, if violent, should be treated first by rubbing the crown of the head with the remedy once, and immediately taking one or two table-spoonsful diluted with hot water ; this should be repeated three or four times each day. The disorder must be very bad if it is not subdued in two or three days ; but perseverance is necessary.

SPRAINS are easily cured with this remedy ; sometimes by merely rubbing ; but if that does not succeed, by taking a long piece of linen, about two inches broad, and wrapping it several times round the part, after it has been saturated with the remedy, they are generally cured in a day or two ; but the linen should be kept moist with the remedy the whole of the time, until a cure is effected.

BRUISES sometimes require to be several times rubbed with the remedy. At other times once or twice suffices: but it is always well to persevere until the cure is effected. The application gives no pain ; but sometimes bruises are rather tedious in being cured.

SCURVY only requires to be rubbed with the remedy several times until the complaint is subdued. But if the person afflicted considers his blood to be any way bad, he will do well to have the crown of the head rubbed with the remedy, and take one or two table-spoonsful, diluted with hot water, each morning before breakfast, for twelve mornings. It will generally purify the blood in that time.

ITCH, I believe, may be cured by this remedy, by washing or rubbing with it till the complaint is subdued. But this is often tedious, and requires perseverance and great cleanliness.

RING-WORMS, upon children's heads, are easily cured by rubbing the head with the remedy. It very seldom takes a week to cure the complaint, and nothing can be done which conduces more to the general health of children than rubbing the head. Many schools are broken up by this teasing complaint, which might be avoided by the master or mistress using it for the children. I believe its infecting qualities are removed by the first application.

PARALYTIC ATTACKS should be attended to the same moment as the attack commences ; and this will show the necessity of all families being provided with a bottle ready prepared. The crown of the head should be well rubbed with the remedy, and at the same time the patient should have two table-spoonsful for a woman, and three table-spoonsful for a man given, diluted with hot water. Another person ought to be employed in rubbing the part affected with the remedy. Perhaps it may be necessary to give the patient more than one dose; but this must be left to the discretion of his friends. It is sure to do good in repeating it.

PREGNANCY.—Pregnant women ought to take one table-spoonful diluted with hot water, once a week or fortnight, but not oftener, during their pregnancy. It renders the child more healthy, and the delivery is effected with greater ease.

BITES OF POISONOUS REPTILES are easily cured by rubbing the parts bitten with the remedy. It neutralises the poison, and heals the sore in a very short time; but it is well to do it immediately after the bite has been given.

BITES OF MAD DOGS, or any other dogs, are easily cured by rubbing well the part bitten with this remedy. I believe no uneasiness may be felt by the person bitten, if it is rubbed the same day; but it is always best to do it immediately after, and it ought to be rubbed several times, and a piece of soft linen, saturated with the remedy, applied to the part. This is one of those cases which I have not proved by fact, not having come under my notice; and I have not had occasion to prove it upon myself.

STINGS OF WASPS, BEES, &c., are cured by rubbing the part immediately after being stung; the relief, as well as the attack, is instantaneous; but I do not think it does much good if the part is suffered to swell; therefore the application should be prompt.

ERISIPELAS is cured by rubbing the part with the remedy. A clergyman in the North has had the kindness to communicate a case which I will give in his own words:— "The patient was a woman. Having occasion to call at the house on business, one morning about ten o'clock, I found the poor creature more dead than alive, from violent pain, and a sensation of burning heat in her arms and hands, which were red with inflammation from the fingers to the elbows. She was in perfect misery, she said, having been unable to sleep a moment for two nights. Some aperient medicine had been given her, but there had been no external application to the parts affected. I asked her if I might try to relieve her;—she replied, I might do anything I liked. Accordingly, with this permission, I sent to my house for a cupful of the remedy, which I kept ready prepared; and with this I proceeded to bathe both hands and arms for about ten minutes. The effect was almost miraculous, and the poor creature laughed for joy. This, as I have said, was about ten o'clock, A. M. About noon I called again, to see whether things were going on right, when the patient was fast asleep and comfortable. In the evening she was still better, having bathed herself again. In short in forty-eight hours exactly, the cure was completed. Not only was all pain removed, but the limbs had recovered their usual appearance and every trace of discoloration on the skin had vanished." This will show how much good may be done, with little trouble, by ministers of the Gospel; and it is really part of their work to promote the health of their parishioners and hearers; therefore I hope that all such will make themselves acquainted with the contents of this little publication, and apply them where they may be useful.

Tic Doloreux.—This painful complaint may be greatly relieved by the use of this remedy; perhaps cured if it is in the face. The crown of the head should be well rubbed with the remedy; after which the ear on the side of the head next it should be filled with the remedy, which should remain in for ten minutes. After, the part affected should be rubbed with the remedy. If these fail of effecting a cure, I should recommend that the patient should take two table-spoonsful of the remedy, diluted with hot water, each morning before breakfast, about an hour, for fourteen days.

Scrofula must be very difficult to cure; but as it is in the blood, that ought to be purified, which is easily effected, by first rubbing the crown of the head once with the remedy, after which the patient should take one or two table-spoonsful of the remedy, diluted with hot water, an hour before breakfast, every morning for at least a month; and the sores should be covered with soft linen, saturated with the remedy. It will also be well to apply something softening to the sore. I know of nothing better than tallow. I do not say that this will cure, but I do say that it will alleviate the pain of the sufferer, and change a life of pain and misery to one of comparative comfort and ease.

Bilious Complaints are cured by rubbing first the crown of the head once before retiring to rest, and next morning taking two table-spoonsful of the remedy diluted with hot water, an hour before breakfast, for twenty mornings. Before half of that time is passed the good effects of the application will be seen in the face of the patient, which, from sickly yellow or white, will become fair and ruddy. But this is a small part of the benefit, as the afflicted will acknowledge.

Bites of Musquitoes, Gnats, and other Noxious Insects, may be cured by only rubbing the part bitten with the remedy.

Plague, being an inflammatory complaint, I hope may be cured, by the same method as others of the same description; that is, by first rubbing the crown of the head, and immediately after giving the patient three table-spoonsful, diluted with hot water, which ought to be repeated every ten minutes, if the patient can take it, until the complaint is subdued. I wish this could be introduced into the Turkish empire; many valuable lives would be spared if it were successful, of which I have very little doubt.

Mortification is almost as easily stopped, and the cure effected, if I may judge by the only case which has come under my observation, as any other sore. It was of the person who had his hand crushed by a cart, mentioned in my last year's address, and who had a part of one of his fingers taken off. It was applied as to any common sore, by wrapping a piece of soft linen, saturated with the remedy, upon the sore and kept humid, by wetting it several times a day.

BOILS AND ABSCESSES should be covered with a piece of soft linen, saturated with the remedy, and kept wet. By this means though it does not prevent or retard the bursting of the boil or abscess, it very much relieves the pain by removing the inflammation.

CUTS.—As a tincture, I do not think that this remedy has its equal, giving very little pain when first applied, and curing in a short time. Any person will know that the application should be made by saturating a piece of linen in the remdey, and wrapping it round the part cut, which must be very severe if there is occasion to remove the linen till the cure is effected. But it should be kept always moist by adding a little of the remedy several times each day.

WHITLOW may be cured by either holding the finger in the remedy, or saturating a piece of soft linen with it, and wrapping it round the sore. But it should be kept wet until the cure is effected.

LUMBAGO, though comprised under the head of Rheumatism, it is well to observe, is generally removed by rubbing the part. But if it cannot be removed by that means, or it returns again, I should recommend the patient to have the crown of the head well rubbed once, on retiring to rest, with the remedy, and then taking, for several mornings, an hour before breakfast, two table-spoonsful of the remedy, diluted with hot water.

JAUNDICE, I believe, may be cured by rubbing the crown of the head once, on retiring to rest, and taking two table-spoonsful, diluted with hot water, for several mornings, an hour before breakfast, until the complaint disappears, which I expect it will do in eight or ten days.

LIVER COMPLAINTS AND AFFECTIONS OF THE HEART can only be removed by putting the intestines in a healthful state, which may be effected by rubbing the crown of the head once, on retiring to rest, and each morning taking two table-spoonsful of the remedy, diluted with hot water, an hour before breakfast; perhaps it requires to be taken for months before the complaints are cured. But prevention is always better than cure, therefore the intestines should be kept healthy, and the blood pure.

SORES OF LONG STANDING are relieved, and very often cured, by this remedy, by saturating soft linen with it, and applying it to the sore. After three or four applications it always relieves the pain; and the most obstinate setfasts are removed, and that without pain, in a few days, and the sore becomes clean, not only from that, but all other impurities. How many poor creatures pass lives of misery from incurable sores, who will be relieved by the use of this remedy! There are many instances of persons who have not been able to sleep for weeks, who have slept the very first night after its application; and all, let their case be ever so bad, may have the same consolation if they apply this simple remedy. A gentleman of Hull says, " I found it very efficacious myself, to wet a piece of fine linen with the remedy, and bind it on the diseased part, which I always kept moist, by pouring a few drops upon the linen. The more frequent the application of the remedy the better. This I strictly attended to for three weeks, and though my leg had been bad for months, and bid defiance to the best medical aid I could procure, and caused me to give up all hopes of recovery, to my great surprise the inflammation was entirely gone, the wound was healed, and well in a month."

YELLOW FEVER, which often terminates in the Black Fever, called the Black Vomit, is, I suppose, much of the same nature as the Plague; therefore it must be treated in the same manner. I have no doubt but a great many lives may be preserved by that method.

GALL STONES are no doubt produced by the intestines being in an unhealthy state : therefore it is well to keep them always healthy, which may be generally effected by rubbing the crown of the head once, and taking the remedy, each morning for a week or ten days, an hour before breakfast, diluted with hot water. A beloved sister suffered, and was confined to bed, for several months, by refusing to use it as above. After the Gall Stones are formed, I do not think they can be removed by any other than the ordinary method, but the pain may be greatly alleviated by the application of this remedy ; the pain ought to be attacked in every possible way, by rubbing the exterior, and applying fomentations to the part nearest the pain.

INDIGESTION may be easily corrected by rubbing the crown of the head once, and taking one or two table-spoonsful of the remedy, diluted with hot water, every morning, until the complaint is removed ; as a corrective, this remedy is very efficacious.

SPINAL COMPLAINTS, I believe, have their source in the head ; therefore it will be well first to rub the crown of the head with the remedy, on retiring to rest, after which, next morning, the patient should take one or two table-spoonsful of the remedy, diluted with hot water, an hour before breakfast, each morning, for twelve mornings, or till the complaint is removed. Soft linen, of several thicknesses, saturated with the remedy, should be applied to the part where the pain is, if rubbing does not remove it, and it should be renewed several times a day if the spine is very painful, and always kept moist. Application, in this manner, for two or three days, is sure to reduce the pain, though it may not cure the complaint so soon.

Through Mr. V., of Hull, who has received great benefit himself in the cure of a bad and inflamed leg and rheumatism, I am enabled to add many well authenticated cases; the whole of those persons are now living in his neighbourhood, therefore those benefitted may be seen, and I am given to understand that they will answer any questions which may be put to them:—

1. A Lady at Grimsby cured of rheumatism in the arm.

2. A Gentleman at York cured of violent rheumatism in his hands, which had been of long standing.

3. A Gentleman at Hull cured of lumbago.

4. Two Women were cured of violent sore throats; but they lost their husbands of the same complaint, because they would not use the remedy; they were of that class to whom it does no good.

5. Mrs. Williams, Finkle-street, cured of inflammation in the throat and lungs.

6. Mrs. Harrison, 41 Saville-street, cured of spasms and indigestion.

7. Mr. Craggs, Dock-street, cured of pain in the side.

8. Ann Banks, Myton-street, quite cured of a paralytic stroke, though she had lost the use of one side, called at Mr. Vallance's shop and gave him her own acccount of the cure, which she attributed solely to the remedy of Brandy and Salt. She took as much as **two** glasses full each day.

9. Captain Plumb, of the vessel Ann, Keddy's Wharf, rheumatism in the head and all over the body. He appeared very near death. Mr. V. recommended the Brandy and Salt. He rubbed his head, and took it according to prescription; on the fourth day he called, with a smile on his countenance, and said he was much better. He continued to recover, and is now quite well.

10. Mrs. Hodgson, Myton-Gate, sore throat cured.

11. Mrs. Wardle, Bishop-Lane, violent pain at the heart, who had been unwell for several months, and was given up by three physieiaus. Her complaint was removed in a few weeks, and she is now able to attend to her domestic concerns, though she has a family, and keeps a public house.

12. Mrs. Brown, Labour-in-Vain public house, cured of violent pains in the head.

13. A man at Flambro', cured of a white swelling in the knee. His wife of a bad leg also.

14. Mr. Bealby, cured of a bad leg.

15. Mr. Easton, Hull and Brigg carrier, cured of a bad leg of twenty-two years' standing.

16. James Calvert, Agnes-Place, cured of an abscess in the lungs and consumption.

17. John Crowest, Pilot, Manchester-Place, in the last stage of a consumption, cured. This person and James Calvert applied to Mr. V. at the same time. The application of the remedy caused them to throw off the stomach, by coughing, an immense quantity of cor-

rupt matter, mingled with blood and phlegm, for several nights ; but after it was discharged, their coughs ceased entirely, and they thought themselves quite well. From gratitude they called to thank Mr. V. who went with them to the doctor. He was surprised at the cure, as he thought it an impossibility, their deaths having been considered inevitable. Calvert was cautioned not to take cold, as one half of his lungs was gone. He said, " I never was better in my life, except a little weakness in my legs."

18. —— Robinson, a poor man, very bad of Rheumatism, not able to walk, driven about the streets of Hull in a carriage drawn by two dogs, quite cured in a few weeks, and able to walk and attend to his business.

19. Mrs. Hardy, near Waltham-street Chapel, cured of a large tumour upon the neck.

20. A boy had his foot severely bruised by a shutter falling upon it ; was cured in a week by the application of the remedy.

THOSE TO WHOM IT DOES NO GOOD.—There is a large class in society to whom it does no good—they are those who will not use it ; but I have no doubt they are daily diminishing in number, for after any one has applied it to any complaint, the benefits are so manifest that it would be to suppose them not endowed with common sense not to apply it again in case of need ; it only requires very little reflection to know how to apply it to any complaint, whether external or internal, and there is not the least fear of any bad effects from it. Experience of several years has convinced me that it has never yet done any harm, but its efficacy is much more certain when it is used clear.

INFLAMMATION.—I saw it stated in a newspaper that a professioual gentleman had published a treatise to prove that complaints of all kinds are caused by inflammation ; this coincides with my opinion and observation ; and such being the case, it is not surprising that this remedy has cured almost every complaint to which it has been properly applied, or has greatly relieved them ; but the universality of its efficacy has been thought by some a great objection to it. A lady to whom it was recommended said—" I have no faith in it, for you say that it cures so many complaints ; if you said it cured only one, I could use it for that ; but as you say there are so many, I will not use it for any." This may be wisdom ; but, as I have known it cure the head, ear and tooth-ache, inflammation in the eyes, ague, cholic, pains in the side, chilblains, burns and scalds, cancers, and several other complaints, and some of them scores of times, I should be wanting in my duty if I did not recommend it for them.

CANCERS. It has been applied in six cases of cancer, five of which it has cured, and that without pain ; even the first application did not give pain but relief ; three of these were very severe, and had been of long continuance ; the other two were at the commencement, and to the sixth it was applied but once, which brought on a great bleeding, which I believe, was necessary, as the patient was much better for it; but it alarmed his friends, they called in his medieal advisers, (he being a wealthy man, he had the best the place could afford,) they were much offended by its application, and said they would not come again if he continued to use it; he therefore promised he would not use it again, and I believe he kept his promise, as he died in less than twelve months after; and judging from the others, I have no doubt that he would have been cured if he had not been prevented from applying it. The other five are all poor, and are cured and living at present, or were a short time ago; the rich was not cured, and is dead. I wish this had been otherwise, as he is said to have been a worthy man.

SPRAINS.—Many persons suffer from sprains for months, who might be cured, by fomenting the part with this remedy, in a few days, and some of them in a few hours. I have known several who have suffered for weeks, though under very able doctors, cured in a a very short time with it.

A respectable individual informed me that an acquaintance of his, a commercial traveller, who one evening had unfortunately taken the brandy *without* the salt, happened, as he was ascending a stone staircase, to stumble, and in falling, to bring his head in contact with the edge of one of the steps. In consequence of this, a great portion of the skin was rubbed off his forehead. There being Salted Brandy in the house, he had the courage to apply it to the raw surface! The accident occured on the Friday evening, and the embrocation was continued till Sunday night, and on Monday morning the wound was sufficiently healed to admit of his wearing his hat and entering on his journey.

The Cashier in a gentleman's office in Liverpool accidentally received a very smart blow on the back of his left hand, from the edge of a door opened hastily by one of the workmen, who was not aware that any one stood in the way. The injury was followed by such inflammation as completely deprived him of the use of his fingers. He instantly applied the Salted Brandy, which so reduced the swelling that he obtained the perfect use of his hand in about three hours after he had received the blow. This account I had from his own lips, in the presence of his employer, who confirmed the statement.

A gentleman told me of a case of violent inflammation in the chest, in which he administered a dose of this remedy in the evening, and the following morning found the patient relieved. I was informed that the physician in attendance was not over pleased with my friend having, with the usual kindness of his disposition, and in the simplicity of his heart, interfered on the occasion.

A farm-servant had some swelling on the side of his face, which was probably the Mumps, of such intensity that he could not possibly open his mouth. My advice having been asked by the gentleman who communicated the case, and in whose service he lived, I recommended the Salted Brandy to be given internally, through a quill, in the prescribed dose, twice a day, and a piece of linen, several folds thick, thoroughly saturated with the preparation, to be applied to the tumour, and to be kept constantly moist. This recommendation was complied with on, I believe, the Sunday evening; and his master told me afterwards that the man resumed his work on the following Thursday.

The above instances of the efficacy of Salted Brandy, as a sedative of inflammation, I consider as sufficient in this place, especially as, in this respect, its powers will necessarily be brought under notice in the course of what I shall detail under other heads of injuries and diseases, with all of which it will, more or less, be found to be essentially connected. I would here only further remark, that I am quite convinced that it might be used with the happiest effect in attempts to reduce inflammation attending the fracture and the amputation of limbs.

OPEN SORES.—In all cases coming under this head, such as chapped lips and hands, ulcers and excoriations, this preparation will be found very efficacious in allaying the inflammation, arresting the progress of proud flesh, and in healing the part affected.

A lady told me that the hands of a servant maid and lad in her employ were so chapped that they could not use them. She had recourse to the Salted Brandy, which, after the third or fourth application, so reduced the inflammation, as to restore the use of the fingers, and in a short time it completely healed the sores. A similarly happy effect attended its application to a severely chapped hand of a lady of my acquaintance, to whom I had the pleasure of successfully recommending it.

A brother clergyman had an abscess in his right breast. It had been opened in the month of April, but it continued to discharge matter (though repeated attempts had been made to heal it,) till the following October, when I became acquainted with him, and told me of the obstinacy of the ulcer. I recommended a trial of Salted Brandy, and he very kindly put himself under my care. I therefore directed him to take the remedy internally once a day, and to keep it constantly applied to the wound. He did so, and in the course of three weeks or a month it was perfectly healed.

BRUISES.—A lady residing in the eastern part of Liverpool, informed me that a sailor lad, in the employ of a captain of a vessel belonging to the above port, had the misfortune to bruise one of his fingers so severely that his master thought it would be necessary to have it cut off, lest mortification might ensue, as the inflammation had contiued unabated ever since the accident had happened, which was the period of a fortnight; therefore, on the captain's coming ashore, he asked his wife to what surgeon he should send the boy, either for the amputation or cure of his finger. She replied by desiring him to send the lad to her. He did so. She commenced her operations by washing the bruised finger with the Salted Brandy ; she then enveloped it in several folds of linen, which were saturated with the above preparation, and directed the boy to come to her on the following morning. He came accordingly, and on her asking him how his finger was, he said that the last was the only night since he had met with the injury, in which he had enjoyed any sleep, and that the pain had nearly ceased. She repeated the former treatment, and, having continued it for a few days, succeeded in effecting a perfect cure of this little sufferer's finger.

SPRAINS.—The landlord of a respectable hotel in Liverpool detailed to me the following case : A gentleman who was staying at his house happened to sprain his ancle, and was in consequence unable to move his foot. He caused the injured ancle to be embrocated with Salted Brandy during the remainder of the evening, and received so much benefit from the embrocation, that he was able to go out on business the following morning. Salted Brandy, however, is not only of great service when applied to a sprain immediately on its occurrence, but it is also very beneficial in cases of injured muscles, from sprains long since received.

INDURATED TUMOURS.—The following case was communicated to me by a friend, in the presence of a physician, who was also acquainted with it. A person had an indurated tumour on the back of one of his hands, in consequence, I suppose, (for my friend did not assign the cause which produced it,) of some external injury. The country surgeon completely failing to reduce it, the patient went up to London, where he entrusted the treatment of the tumour to one of the most eminent surgeons there ; but after he had submitted to it for some time, he returned to the country, having experienced no benefit whatever. He again called in the service of his former medical attendant, and, while under his care, he heard of Salted Brandy, and applied it as an embrocation to the part affected. Resolved to give it a fair trial, he entirely discontinued the liniments sent him, and did not tell his surgeon what he was using ; but, after he had tried it for some time, he showed him his hand, and he pronounced it to be advancing towards a cure. The patient then acknowledged what course he had adopted, and being encouraged to persevere in it, he, in a short time afterward, succeeded in completely reducing the tumour and recovering the perfect use of his hand.

A gentleman living in Chester had a nodule or tumour on his face, which very much disfigured it. He perseveringly embrocated it with Salted Brandy, and entirely reduced it.

Ere I quit this part of my subject, I would suggest the probability of Salted Brandy proving efficacious for the reduction of *wens, bronchocele*, or, what is properly called, *goitre.*

PARALYSIS.—A worthy friend of mine told me that he prevailed on an acquaintance of his in Ireland, one of the sides of whose body was so paralyzed that he could neither walk nor do anything else without assistance, to take the Salted Brandy internally, and also to cause the side, of which he had lost the use, to be well rubbed with it twice a day. He commenced this course immediately; and my friend happening to call on him about a week afterwards, found his patient, to his great but agreeable surprise, hobbling about unattended in his garden.

RHEUMATISM.—A military captain, residing in Liverpool, to whom I was introduced, was so afflicted with rheumatism as to be confined to his bed. He had availed himself of the services of the faculty, and had applied various embrocations, but with no decided benefit. He complained of being very weak in body. This I could easily believe; because rheumatism of itself will cause much debility, and as the strong sudorific medicines which are generally administered in this disorder, as well as those of a drastic nature, cause much exhaustion, and, consequently, weakness, there can be no doubt of a rheumatic subject being weakened by the ordinary course of medical treatment. I talked to him about Salted Brandy, and succeeded in persuading him to take it inwardly, and to apply it externally to the parts affected. The happy result was that, in the course of three weeks, he was enabled to rise from his bed and to use his right hand, with which he had not been able to write for several years previously, and he was considerably improved in his general health.

I have it in my power to communicate several other cases of rheumatic subjects whose limbs have been restored to their usual offices, and whose health has been greatly benefited by their taking this medicine; but I consider the case above detailed to be sufficient evidence in favor of the salutary effect of Salted Brandy in rheumatism, whether chronic or acute—whether affecting the hip joint, and then given the appellation of *sciatica*, or the region of the loins, and therefore called *lumbago*. It may be right also to remark, that this remedy might be used with, perhaps, good effect in cases of stiff knees, and other joints similarly affected.

ERYSIPELAS.—The case of a complete cure of erysipelas was lately communicated to me by a friend, whose brother was the individual troubled with it. The seat of the disease was the leg, (it being that kind of erysipelas which is confined to an affection of the skin, but which does not pervade the system,) and it had been of two years' standing. Its progress had been formerly arrested by other remedies; the enemy, however, was not subdued, but was only repulsed for a season. It would return after a time, and would renew its ravages; and a total defeat of the foe and a complete cure of the disease were not accomplished, until the Salted Brandy had been internally taken, and, at the same time, had been externally applied.

I have successfully administered it to little children not seven years of age, who were laboring under the effects of this distressing disorder.

JAUNDICE.—This is a most unpleasant malady; and the method adopted for its removal, namely, a course of smart and continued purgation, is not only tedious, but calculated to weaken the body, and in some kinds, or rather stages, of this complaint, to endanger the life of the patient, not as a direct but as an indirect consequence, because the above treatment renders the body (especially when under the effect of blue pill, frequently, but, I think, very improperly given in this disease) very susceptible of cold; and cold caught in the jaundice has not unfrequently been the cause of death. But the patient need have very little apprehension of taking cold while under a course of Salted Brandy; because this medicine, though acting as a powerful diaphoretic, makes the body less susceptible of cold than it is otherwise, and especially when affected by drastic medicines.

About four years ago, I had a very severe attack of jaundice, of which I was not cured by the ordinary mode of treatment in less than two months' time. I relapsed into the disorder every subsequent spring and autumn, and I had recourse to the same medicine as had at first removed it. I continued subject to these relapses till the autumn of the year 1839, when I found my health worse than ever I knew it to be from the effects of this sickly and enervating disease; and, having persevered in the use of several remedies prescribed for its restoration, and finding it still unimproved, I began to despair of long surviving such a state of illness as I then experienced.

Happening one day to be in the office of a friend in Liverpool, one of his oldest servants, having observed to me how ill I appeared, asked (on my answering that I was very ill, and that I could not meet with anything which would cure me) whether I had ever heard of Brandy and Salt? I said that I had heard of such a preparation, but that I had no more faith in it than in ditch water. He then told me that he had been labouring under tightness in the chest, a sore throat, and an inflammation in the bowels, all at once, and that the Salted Brandy had cured him of all the three. This was my first introduction to this remedy, and the above report induced me to make a trial of its powers. I immediately commenced taking it; yet I was not actuated on the occasion by any confidence I had in its efficacy, for I felt not any. I persevered, however, in using it, (though I cherished no other hope of its curing me than a drowning man really has of his being saved from a watery grave when he catches at a straw,) and in the course of a fortnight I found that I was completely set to rights, the liver doing its duty, and my health and spirits entirely restored. As, however, I expected a relapse in the ensuing November, in which in the year preceding, I had sustained an attack, I continued to take the remedy till the expiration of that month. In order to be clearly understood, I ought to state that, from November

1838, till the period of my being cured, in 1839, I was almost constantly subject to the disorder; yet, November being the month in
which I used periodically to relapse, I considered it advisable to con-
tinue taking the Salted Brandy in order to break the force of an attack, in case I should again sustain one; but I experienced no relapse in November, and continued, till the beginning of July free
from the effects of the disease, and was enabled to pass the whole of
the winter without putting on a great coat, which I had been constantly obliged to wear for the previous fourteen years of my life.
In the beginning of last July I relapsed again; but having again had
recourse to this medicine, I had not to wait a month or five weeks
for my recovery, but I was restored to perfect convalescence in eight
or nine days' time.

Having received so much benefit from this medicine, so providen-
tially brought under my notice, I considered that it was my duty, after
I had obtained all the information within my reach, and had, to the
best of my ability, reasoned respecting it, to recommend it to others.
I had not long to wait for an opportunity of so doing, for a very excellent young man, a member of the congregation to which I had the
privilege of a share in ministering, was, shortly after my own recovery, attacked with jaundice. I prescribed him Salted Brandy, and
thereby cured him *in five days!* To another individual, a tailor, who
had labored under this disorder for a very long time, and had deriv-
ed no benefit from the usual mode of treatment, this remedy was
recommended by a friend of mine. At first he was quite disinclined
but was subsequently persuaded to try it. In his case, which was a
very inveterate one, its operation was very slow; but it eventually
proved to be sure.

INDIGESTION.—It will be sufficient, under this head, to observe
that I have ample grounds for asserting that a more speedily effica-
cions medicine than Salted Brandy cannot be administered for the
removal of dispepsia, or indigestion.

HEART-BURN.—This is an unpleasant heat or burning sensation
in the stomach, and will be much sooner and more effectually corrected by Salted Brandy, than either by carbonate of soda or magnesia.

SPASMS.—A great variety of nervous disorders comes under this
head; but, as this work is written more especially for the use of the
lower classes of society than for the edification or entertainment of
the learned, and so puts forth no pretensions to a scientific or professional treatise, the word used as an introduction or heading to this
paragraph, is to be taken in the commonly received acceptation of it.

A lady, who was staying in Liverpool a short time, and had apart-
ments in the house in which I lodged, was subject to such violent
spasms as occasionally produced alarming apprehensions. The land-
lady told her of the Salted Brandy, and of the great benefit which
I and others had received from taking it. She in consequence re-

quested an interview with me, which I felt most happy to afford her. I prevailed on her to try this medicine, and I mixed her a bottle of it, which she took with her. In the course of three weeks or a month after she had joined her family, her husband wrote to a common friend to say of what essential service the Salted Brandy had been to her, and to request the transmission of the newspaper which contained an account respecting it, with a view to the dissemination of the knowledge of this extraordinary and excellent remedy in his parts of the kingdom. In the cholic, also, it will be found most serviceable.

PALPITATION OF THE HEART.—In this disease the medicine in question, or rather beyond all question, will be found very serviceable. It should be taken internally, as well as externally applied to the part affected.

NETTLE-RASH.—I cured a lad of about thirteen years of age, who was labouring under this complaint, with Salted Brandy. It was taken internally; and its application to the wheals or bumps, which sometimes (and did in this case) accompany this disease, and are attended with a very troublesome itching, caused them in a very short time to subside, and the itching to cease entirely.

FITS, WHETHER HYSTERIC OR EPILEPTIC.—To a young lady, who was very subject to fits, I prescribed the Salted Brandy. She took it for a fortnight or three weeks, and experienced, not only a cessation of these attacks, but a decided improvement in her general health; and she continued for several months free from the recurrence of a single fit.

I also heard of this medicine having been administered with promise of success in the case of a gentleman who used to be seized by several epileptic fits in the course of the day.

DYSENTERY.—A friend informed me that the master of a vessel belonging to Liverpool cured several of his crew, who had been attacked with dysentery at Havana. He also cured, by means of the same medicine, two fellow master-mariners; one of whom, a young man, was alarmingly ill. This gentleman says that he needs no other remedy in his medicine chest save Salted Brandy.

ASTHMA.—Another friend communicated to me the case of a respectable farmer in Cheshire, who laboured under the effects of this disease to such a degree, that he was obliged to sleep in an erect posture, having been enabled, after taking a pint of Salted Brandy, in the prescribed doses, to lie down to rest without inconvenience.

The principal of a respectable firm in the corn trade in Liverpool, who had for many years suffered from an obstinate asthma, was induced to try Salted Brandy for its removal. He made the preparation accordingly, and took the dose in the manner prescribed, and

c

he very soon experienced great benefit from the medicine. This individual spoke in the highest terms of its virtues, and wished that they might be universally known.

CHOLERA MORBUS.—I have been creditably informed that Salted Brandy proved quite a specific in the above awful disorder; and I feel perfectly convinced that not only in this, but in every other inflammatory and spasmodic complaint, this remedy may be used with the greatest safety and the most beneficial results. In my own case, I took the prescribed dose three times in one day for a violent inflammation with which I was attacked in the bowels, and completely succeeded in a short time in stopping the diarrhœa, and in allaying the pain; which was a sure sign of my having subdued the inflammation.

CANCER.—I know of a case of this disorder having been cured, by the exhibition of Salted Brandy, in a woman who is nearly sixty years of age, and on whom the operation of the excision of the diseased breast had been performed, but to no purpose; for, after the wound had been healed up, she was professionally informed that the cancer had not been eradicated, and that to effect its entire removal a second operation would be necessary. Subsequently to her having been sent home from the Infirmary, she became so much worse, and was apparently so near her death, that she was prayed for in the church; about which time a neighbor told her of Salted Brandy, as reported to have proved efficacious in curing cancer, and recommended her to try it. She did so, and in the course of eight or nine days from her having commenced using this medicine, which she took internally twice a day, and kept constantly applied to the part affected with pain, by means of a piece of folded linen saturated with the preparation—in the course, I say, of eight or nine days, she told me that she experienced what she had not felt for twenty years previously, namely, an appetite for food. She daily improved in health and strength, and she appeared, the last time I saw her, to have taken, as the saying is, a new lease of her life!

Another woman residing not far distant from the village in which lives the subject of the above notice, and having a cancer in her breast, has found considerable benefit from the use of the remedy in question. When she began taking it, she could neither eat nor sleep well; but within a fortnight of her having commenced this course of medicine, she recovered her appetite and enjoyed sound sleep. She informed me that, a short time before she was advised to try this remedy, leeches had been applied to her breast, but that they could get very little blood, the color of which was very unhealthy; but that upon her again applying them, in about ten days after she had commenced using the Salted Brandy, they drew the blood copiously, and that its color was greatly improved. Her husband said that, during the forty years in which he and his wife had lived together, he had never known her sensibly perspire; but that she perspired profusely after she had for some days used the Salted Brandy. From the foregoing communication I ascertained these two particulars, namely, that this medicine tends, as I had maintained previously, to purify the blood, and acts as a powerful diaphoretic.

TOOTHACHE.—A respected friend communicated to me a case wherein Salted Brandy had proved of essential service in allaying the agony of this distractingly painful affection. In, however, cases of pain supposed to arise from a carious tooth, I would caution the patient against too readily concluding that the pain proceeds from the nerve of a decayed tooth; because, in many instances, violent pain in the maxillary part of the face, in persons of delicate fibre, and women, during the period of pregnancy, has been known to exist where no defect in any tooth was the exciting cause. The teeth are such important instruments, that I would advise every person suffering from pain in the region of the jaws, and supposing that it must arise from a decayed tooth, to obtain the clearest proof that such is the cause of the painful affection, ere the resolution be taken to have the tooth extracted. Before I take leave of this head, I would observe that the soundness of the teeth may be best secured, and, in consequence, much pain avoided, by cleaning them with a brush and cold water just before bed-time; and that, if the pain in the face should proceed from some other cause than that of cariousness in any tooth, I would dissuade patients from using those narcotic preparations so generally recommended and unfortunately adopted for tic-doloreux, and similar affections; because such remedies often prove more prejudicial than the evil which they are intended to remove; for, instead of curing, they lay the foundation of fresh suffering, and not unfrequently render the cure ultimately impracticable. The course, therefore, which I would recommend the patient to pursue, should be an attempt to strengthen the system by avoiding every thing having a tendency to induce debility, taking Salted Brandy internally for a couple of months at a time, and using, if practicable, as much exercise in the open air as possible. This, I believe, will be found the most effectual means of removing pains in the face or elsewhere, originating in nervous debility.

SORE-THROAT.—I have had frequent opportunities of proving the efficacy of Salted Brandy in this complaint. It should be used in its undiluted state as a gargle, and as an embrocation to that part of the throat where the inflammation appears to be seated. Its effect will be considered truly surprising, if other patients should experience the same immediate benefit from it which I have received in the case of sore-throat. My throat has been so inflamed, about an hour before I went to preach, that deglutition was most painful; yet within that hour, I have succeeded, by gargling and embrocating with Salted Brandy, in entirely reducing the inflammation. Almost similar success has attended the use of this sedative by a very worthy friend of mine, who has been occasionally troubled with soreness of the throat.

PILES.—A case was lately communicated to me in which this medicine had been of signal service in affording relief. In this instance, as well as in all others of an inflammatory character, no error can be committed by using the remedy both internally and locally at the same time.

PULMONARY CONSUMPTION.—A lady favored me with the communication of the following case. She said that her servant maid had such a distressing cough, such profuse perspirations, and such other symptoms of a consumption, that she contemplated expressing, in as delicate a manner as possible, her apprehensions to the poor girl, and recommending her to go home to her parents; but that, happening, when she was on the point of adopting the above course, to hear of the Salted Brandy as much talked of for the cure of this insidious and flattering disorder, she thought she would try it and await the result, before she should take any farther steps. The consequence was, that the young woman soon experienced benefit from its use. The cough ceased, her health was entirely restored, and she is still in this lady's service.

Subsequently to my having written the foregoing case, my attention was directed by a respectable friend to the following statement, which appeared in the *Northumberland Advertiser.*

"BRANDY AND SALT.—A most remarkable cure has been effected of a decided case of cousumption, in the last stage, at Barnardscastle, in the person of Mr. Thomas Thompson, whitesmith, by the use of Brandy and Salt. Mr. T. has been for many months attended by one of the first surgeons in the above town, and had gradually become worse, till there remained by his family no hopes of his amendment: he, however, had recourse, lately, to Brandy and Salt, and he is now as strong as ever he was in his life." I have it in my power to produce several other well authenticated cases of the cure of pulmonary consumption by this remedy.

LIVER COMPLAINT.—A person in the employ of a friend of mine in Liverpool had been for some time in ill health, and in consequence was obliged to leave his work for three months, in order to see what benefit he might receive from medical aid and a change of air. The former, of which he had the advantage for about two months, was the means of partially restoring his health: but in a few weeks afterwards he had a relapse into his old complaint, and he was forced at intervals to leave off working. About this period I became acquainted with the very indifferent state of his health. He looked wretchedly ill, and appeared to be rapidly wasting away. I strongly advised and prevailed on him to try Salted Brandy. At first it made him so sick at stomach, that he was afraid to repeat the dose; but upon my saying that I was glad it had acted as an emetic, and that I was confident that the sickness would shortly cease and no injurious consequences ensue, he again commenced taking the medicine I had recommended. In the course of a fortnight he experienced considerable benefit, manifested in the improved appearance of his countenance, in the restoration of his health, and freedom from pain. He now seems to be quite well; at all events he has not been under the necessity, for the last eleven months, of leaving his work for more than a very few days, on account of ill health.

AFFECTION OF THE URETER.—A respectable man of the name of Peter Shaw, residing in Liverpool, personally communicated to me the following case, which I detail under the above head, being at a loss for any other designation of it. His case was this. He used to be occasionally seized with a most intolerable pain in the left loin. This he had suffered for thirty-three years! For a great length of time he had been under medical treatment; from which, however, failing to obtain any relief of his sufferings, he had at last recourse to Salted Brandy. He did not apply it externally over the part where existed, as was supposed, the cause of the pain, but he took it only internally, and he assured me that it produced the happiest effect; for in one month it proved the means of completely removing the pain with which he had for so many years been so grievously afflicted. As he seemed to wish that his name should appear in connection with the statement of his case, I allowed myself in this one instance to deviate from my original design, which was to give no names of persons whom I reported as having received benefit from the use of Salted Brandy, deeming such a course perfectly unnecessary.

DIABETES.—A case of this nature was communicated to me as having been successfully treated by the use of Salted Brandy, from a quarter which could leave no doubt on my mind as to the cure having been effected by this medicine; for the experiment was made by a professional gentleman on my suggestion.

COLDS.—What is popularly called a cold, is nothing else but a mild species of, or an infant fever, which, if not immediately put to death by *starvation*, may so rapidly attain maturity and such strength, that its expulsion and execution may prove a very difficult and possibly a doubtful matter. "*Stuff a cold and starve a fever*," is a proverb which has been perverted from its original form and import, by those to whom pampering the stomach was a greater concern than the preservation of the health, and it seemed soon enough to give over their gluttony when the cold had begun to assume the serious appearance of a fever; in all probability the above proverb originally was, or ought by right to be, *If you stuff a cold, you will have to starve a fever*; which evidently implies, that indulgence to a cold would terminate in a fever, which nothing short of the most determined exertions and self-denial would be able to subdue and extinguish. I have purposely dilated on the subject of colds, because from them may be dated the rise of a great many diseases which send thousands into eternity, ere they have lived out half the number of their days on earth! Salted Brandy will generally be found most efficacious in removing a cold, whether it be confined more particularly to the head or to the chest, or whether it pervade the whole body, by allaying the inflammation, and restoring to the obstructed perspiration a free passage through its accustomed channels.

SICKNESS AT STOMACH.—Salted Brandy will be attended with very good effect in cases of nausea or disordered stomach; and might, therefore, prove highly beneficial to pregnant women, who are generally troubled in the above manner during some, or the greater part, of the period of gestation. I know of its speedy effect in removing nausea; but as this is a *nauseous* subject, I shall not enter into any detail of cases, nor offer any further remarks on it, except to suggest the possibility, (can I venture to add the probability?) of this preparation being of service to the patient seized with *Sea-sickness!*

" SCROFULA.—A highly respectable and much esteemed friend communicated to me the efficacy of Salted Brandy in this disease. " We gave," says he, " the remains of a bottle of this mixture to a poor woman laboring under scrofulous affections, last spring. She is perfectly cured."

The following observations are extracted from a recent publication :

"Many entertain a prejudice against the use of Brandy as a medicine, and so do I; but the Brandy is a very different thing taken by itself, from what it is when impregnated with Salt. As I never take ardent spirits, and my general beverage is water, what I am about to state may be considered worthy the greater attention. For the sake of experiment, I have taken two table-spoonsful of Brandy in as much hot water, and the consequence was a most unpleasant burning sensation in my stomach and flush in my face; whereas no such result followed the prescribed dose of medicine in question, nor did I feel, after the lapse of a minute from taking it, as if I had received ardent spirits into my stomach; whence I concluded that the Salt had such an effect on the Brandy as to remove the usual deleterious effect of the ardent spirit.

" Some medical gentlemen have, but with all due deference I think without proper consideration, cautioned their patients against the preparation in question, on the ground of its liability to produce inflammation; but it appears to me most surprising that it should be productive of *internal* inflammation, seeing that, when applied as an *embrocation* it acts as a most powerful and speedy sedative; and that such it proves in cases of internal as well as external inflammation, is evident from its wonderful efficacy as a gargle for a sore throat. These gentlemen hesitate not to prescribe Brandy and Water, sweetened with sugar, as a tonic to very weak patients: why, therefore, should they consider diluted Brandy and Salt so dangerous, the alteration being the substitution of Salt instead of the sugar? If this preparation has an imflammatory tendency, let them prove that it has this effect; but I believe that they would not enter the lists with me in this contest. The diluted Brandy and Salt has over the diluted Brandy and Sugar not only a medical but a moral advantage; because a too great fondness may be engendered for the latter, while there need be no apprehensions whatever that such a habit for the former will ever be contracted, notwithstanding the old proveıb, that habit is a second nature, and the force of acquired tastes.

"As I purpose taking a future opportunity, should my life be spared, of entering more fully into detail on the subject of this excellent medicine, I shall close these remarks by recommending to those who may be induced to take it, *perseverance* in its use, and the total discontinuance of that mode of living which has a tendency to foster the malady, for the removal of which they have recourse to this preparation; and that as God is as well the preserver and restorer of our health as he is the author of our being, and effects his purposes by the intervention of means, no one should use this or any other medicine either superstitiously on the one hand, or irreligiously on tle other; but in dependence on the Deity for his blessing, and in entire resignation to his will as to the result."

Boston, 7 Nov., 1851.

Liberty has been granted to refer to the following gentlemen, who will give information in regard to various cures which have been effected by the use of Brandy and Salt, as herein prescribed.

H. S. BRADLEY, Haverhill, Mass. He had an affection of one of his eyes ; had been to the Eye Infirmary, and received more relief from Salted Brandy than any other medicine.

SAMUEL BIGELOW, of Cambridge, was relieved in a case of vertigo. His daughter also had a very troublesome cough, which was removed by the use of this remedy.

JOHN BENSON, Boston, was afflicted with dispepsia, inflammatory rheumatism and vertigo. Has also used it successfully for diarrhœa and dysentery, burns, scalds, and inflammation generally. Has found it very beneficial in all such cases.

RICHARD WARD, teller in the Atlantic Bank, can give more information in regard to the good effects of Salted Brandy, than any other person in this vicinity.

HUNDREDS OF INDIVIDUALS, who have experienced relief in numerous cases of disease, can testify to the inestimable value of Salted Brandy, as a simple, safe and efficacious remedy.

INDEX.

☞ This pamphlet may be purchased of C. C. P. MOODY, No. 52 Washington Street, Boston.

Printed by BoD™in Norderstedt, Germany